TURNING MONTHS INTO YEARS WORKBOOK

DIANA WRIGHT

Doctor of Naturopathy
B.S.N., M.B.A., N.E.A.-B.C., A.A.D.P.-B.C.

ILLUSTRATED BY TAISA PALMEIRA

ISBN 978-1-7372784-2-9

For more information, address: diana@dianawrightnd.com

First paperback edition April 2021.

Book design by Taisa O. Palmeira

Check out Diana's website: www.dianawrightnd.com.

LEGAL NOTICE:

The information provided in this book is intended to complement what you learned in the *Turning Months into Years* book. It is not a substitute for examination, diagnosis, and medical care provided by a licensed and qualified health professional. If you believe you or your child or someone you know suffer from the conditions described herein, please see your health care provider. Do not attempt to treat yourself, your child, or anyone else without proper medical supervision.

DISCLAIMER OF LIABILITY:

The materials in this book are provided to you "as is" without warranty of any kind, either expressed or implied, including, but not limited to, the implied warranties of merchantability, fitness for a particular purpose, or non-infringement.

My belief is that the body is stressed with an accumulation of environmental and internal factors that prevents the body from healing. As these factors are removed from the body, the body can heal itself as God intended.

In no event shall Diana Wright, her staff, heirs, or assigns nor Private Membership Association, nor Divine Health or their associates or employees be liable for any damages or incidental damages or damages for loss of profits, revenue, use or data, whether brought in contract or tort, arising out of, or connected with this book or the use, reliance upon, or performance of any material contained in or accessed from this book or our website.

Your reading of this book implies that you agree to the legal notice and liability noted above.

DIANA'S STORY

In June 2012 I was diagnosed with Stage IV, ovarian cancer and given 8 months to live. I had visited 6 different physicians and they all failed to correctly diagnose me even though I had 45 appointments with them. The consensus was that I was not handling menopause well. I was seeing an Oncology Gynecologist, an Infection Control doctor, a hormone specialist (because I wanted to rule out the menopause theory) a general practitioner, an internal medicine doctor and a naturopath. The only one who had a clue I was suffering from a female problem was the naturopath.

The cancer was finally diagnosed when I was hospitalized for chest pain and told I had esophageal spasms. I knew that this diagnosis was incorrect. I insisted on having an EGD to rule out this misdiagnosis as it would follow me through my medical records. I needed to know why I was getting sicker every day. Since I was scheduled to have the EGD under sedation, I also scheduled my colonoscopy that was not due for 3 more years. The tumors were seen on the colonoscopy.

My Oncology Gynecologist, who I never saw again, decided to lie to me about the results of the scan in front of 5 of my family members. The next day, when I obtained the results of the tests, I was surprised to realize that the MD I had seen for six years, had downplayed the diagnosis until it was a complete fabrication. He said I would have a small incision and he would not even cut the tumor; he would just pull it away with his hand. Sounds good doesn't it? But how do you remove multiple highly vascularized tumors without cutting them? The answer is that you do not. You spread them throughout the abdominal cavity.

The CAT-Scan showed tumors of the rectum, colon, both ovaries, uterus, and the omentum. It failed to show the tumors that were located on the aorta and vena cava because the scan did not visualize my heart. Had I allowed the MD to operate the doctor at MD Anderson said I would have never gotten off the operating room table.

I immediately went to MD Anderson. I had the worst MD there as fate would have it. She refused to answer any questions except to blame the potential lack of response to chemo on "My tumor has to respond and if it doesn't there was nothing she could do". She would then bolt from the room without answering any questions. This was prior to starting chemo so she did not really expect the chemo to be successful against the tumors. I knew I had to get away from her as she would make my death her priority. There was no way I was going to allow this physician to operate on me when she was telling herself I was dying. I knew her internal spirit would lead her to make mistakes and ultimately lead to my death.

On 2005, I had the flu and could not recover after multiple doctor visits. I had visited the naturopath and an old Chinese health food store owner who got me on the road to health. I knew supplements worked to build up the immune system. I also knew there were some additional treatments available other than chemotherapy, surgery, and radiation. Chemotherapy, surgery, and radiation have a poor statistical prognosis for Stage IV patients.

I began to research. This is my strength. I spent two months researching cancer when one of my dear friends, Jan Steele, found Dr. Ralf Kleef in Vienna, Austria. Dr. Kleef is an Integrative Oncologist who uses a combination of traditional and naturopathic medication and treatments for his patients. He combines good common sense with his medicine, and he makes each patient feel as though they are very important to him. I knew I had made the right decision to leave MD Anderson when at the end of my first interview with Dr. Kleef he grabbed both my hands in his and said, "Mrs. Wright, I am begging you to get well!" Dr. Kleef was trained in America. He has since moved to Budapest, Hungary.

Dr. Kleef showed David and I many kindnesses. He had his own stepson, Marco drive us 5 hours away to Ulm, Germany for surgery. When I was released, he sent Marco to bring me back to Vienna. I do not know how I could have taken a train as weak as I was. I only weighed 108 pounds when I was released from the hospital. I had lost 33 pounds in 4 months.

As of this writing September 2015, my CA 125 is 2.3 and my scans are clear. My results speak for themselves. I still do two IVs per week, take multiple shots, supplements, my diet, and drink a little red wine (part of the therapy for BRCA1).

I am writing this book for my two daughters, Dana, and Julia. During this journey, I discovered I was BRCA 1. Both of my daughters share my diagnosis. I feel that they may need a future of chronologically detailed resources of what I did to beat this horrible disease, survive and come out of Stage IV "free of disease".* They need a resource to follow.

I am not a medical doctor; I am a doctor of naturopathy. Please understand that I am not offering diagnosis, prognosis, treatment, or care. I am sharing my journey as a former cancer patient of my own personal cancer experience. Any medical decision that you choose to make are strictly your own decisions. I recommend you research every topic yourself and see if it makes sense to add this to your pursuit of wellness. I would not implement any treatment until I discussed it with my oncologist. I personally discuss everything with my three oncologists. If you cannot tell your physician what you are doing you have the wrong doctor. Remember this is your life!

*I do not believe that a person is truly ever "Cancer Free", especially when a genetic mutation like BRCA exists. I believe that cancer cells can be beaten back like the weeds in a garden, but they still exist. I believe that the cancer patient has a chance to recover when there are more healthy negative cells with less positive cancer cells, the body is alkaline, has optimal probiotics with decreased inflammation, and a good team of practitioners. Good Luck!

BEGINNING THE CANCER JOURNEY WITH THE RIGHT ATTITUDE

GOD, JESUS, AND THE HOLY SPIRIT

So do not fear, for I am with you; do not be dismayed, for I am your God. I will strengthen you and help you; I will uphold you with my righteous right hand. – Isaiah 41:10

Cancer is not fair. Whatever hopes and dreams we have for our lives must be put on hold when we receive a cancer diagnosis. It is a disease that brings many gifts. When I was first told this, it was hard to understand. But many people give and do many things for you that help you on this journey.

God did not give you cancer. God only gives good things. Many people ask, "Why me?" Could you in good conscience ask to pass this terrible disease on to someone else? To see someone else's life touched by your pain and suffering helps you understand why you had cancer in the first place.

Cancer is hard to deal with emotionally. The negative emotions experienced create an acidic environment which allows cancer to grow. When God is involved and enters your life, gratitude creates an alkaline body environment that is inhospitable to cancer. Cancer does not grow well in an alkaline environment. Let's make it as hard as possible for cancer to grow. Pray. Pray big, pray hard and pray a lot.

Proverbs 17:22 – *A cheerful heart is good medicine,*
but a crushed spirit dries up the bones.

Battling cancer requires a high degree of internal fortitude. You must have a strategy and a plan, execute it, and then reach deep down into yourself and decide that you really want to get well.

Next, decide you will do whatever it takes to get well. Decide that you will follow whatever plan will make a difference in giving your body the very best chances. Make a covenant with God! You will have to give yourself a shot possibly, drink foul tasting concoctions and devote time and money to getting well. You are your own boss, in charge of your own medical treatment and not a spectator on the sidelines. You decide how you live.

Forgive everyone for everything. Say: "I forgive everyone. I can, I do, and I will."

Handle every day and every problem with prayer or meditation. Be grateful! To give yourself internal fortitude you must ask for the grace to make the decisions you must make. Execute the list of actions it takes to control cancer and then give thanks for the gifts you have received.

Who do you need to forgive?

What steps are you going to take to start your forgiveness process?

Remember: If you are not doing anything to stop the cancer, you are doing something to help it grow.
Do not feed the Beast. Do not eat sugar.

Always give thanks for your strength. Ask God for wisdom, guidance, and strength. Thank God every day for healing you from this cancer. Visualize yourself as a small child holding out your hands to our Father God and asking for a complete healing.

What can you be grateful for today?

What can you do today to fill your spirit?

> Handle every day and every problem with prayer or meditation. Be grateful! To give yourself internal fortitude you must ask for the grace to make the decisions you must make. Execute the list of actions it takes to control cancer and then give thanks for the gifts you have received.

STRENGTHENING THE IMMUNE SYSTEM

DIET: A diet of 80% fresh vegetables and juice, whole grains, seeds, nuts, and a little fruit help put the body into an alkaline state. 20% can be from cooked food, including beans. Fresh vegetable juices provide live enzymes that are easily absorbed and get down to cellular levels within 15 minutes to nourish and enhance the growth of healthy cells.

INCREASE: To obtain live enzymes for building healthy cells try drinking fresh vegetable juice (most vegetables, including bean sprouts) and eat some raw vegetables 2 or 3 times a day. Enzymes are destroyed at temperatures of 104 degrees F (40 degrees C), so do not cook them, or, if you do, use low-heat cookware to preserve enzymes.[2]

NCLUDE: Supplements that will strengthen the immune system, such as vitamin D.

AVOID: Sugar substitutes like NutraSweet, Equal, or Spoonful, made with aspartame, which is harmful.

INSTEAD: A better natural substitute would be coconut sugar, manuka honey or molasses, but only in very small amounts, as sugar aids in the growth of cancer. With pancreatic cancer, all sugar will cause it to grow, especially fructose from fruit.

AVOID: Table salt which has a chemical added to bleach it white.

INSTEAD: A better alternative is Bragg's Liquid Aminos or Celtic or Himalayan salt.

AVOID: Milk causes the body to produce mucus in the gastro-intestinal tract. Dairy products contain high levels of growth hormones and antibiotics. Dairy producers have been fed a diet of corn, a Genetically Modified Organism (GMO), which kills all friendly bacteria in the gut, a lack of which weakens the immune system and overall brain health. Cancer feeds on mucus.

INSTEAD: Substitute unsweetened coconut, flax, or almond milk so no mucus is produced. Substitute unsweetened soymilk if you have prostate cancer or can be sure that it is unadulterated, and hormone free so no mucus is produced.

AVOID: Eating a meat-based diet (cancer cells thrive in an acidic environment). Meat also contains livestock antibiotics, growth hormones and parasites, which are all harmful, especially to people with cancer. Meat protein is difficult to digest and requires a lot of digestive enzymes. Undigested meat remaining in the intestines becomes putrefied and leads to more toxic buildup.

INSTEAD: Eat fish, and a little white meat, like chicken.

> “For maximum Immune System Support: Supplement your body with large amounts of vitamin C (10 Grams), and Beta glucans as directed.”

Health cell walls are made of two layers off fat. Cancer cell walls have a tough protein covering. By refraining from or reducing your consumption of meat, more enzymes are freed to attack the protein walls of cancer cells and allow the body's killer cells to destroy the cancer cells.

What steps are you going to take to strengthen your immune system?

Remember: If you are not doing anything to stop the cancer, you are doing something to help it grow.
Do not feed the Beast. Do not eat sugar.

THE LANGUAGE OF ENERGY

"He gives strength to the weary and increases the power of the weak." - Isaiah 40:29

The Wright Focus: The body can heal itself if there is a properly functioning immune system at the same time decreasing body stress while providing the body with the correct pH, voltage, and raw materials necessary to make new cells while eliminating toxins and infections that will damage the new cells.

There are many things both in our environment and by the lifestyles we live that put stress on the body. When enough stress occurs, the energy frequency drops, and disease starts. The immune system gets confused on what disease is the priority and often focuses on trying to heal the easiest one first. The Wright focus is to remove as many things as possible that causes stress to increase.

When you first saw the energy frequency of emotions chart, what were your thoughts? Did you know how intensely your emotions affected your body?

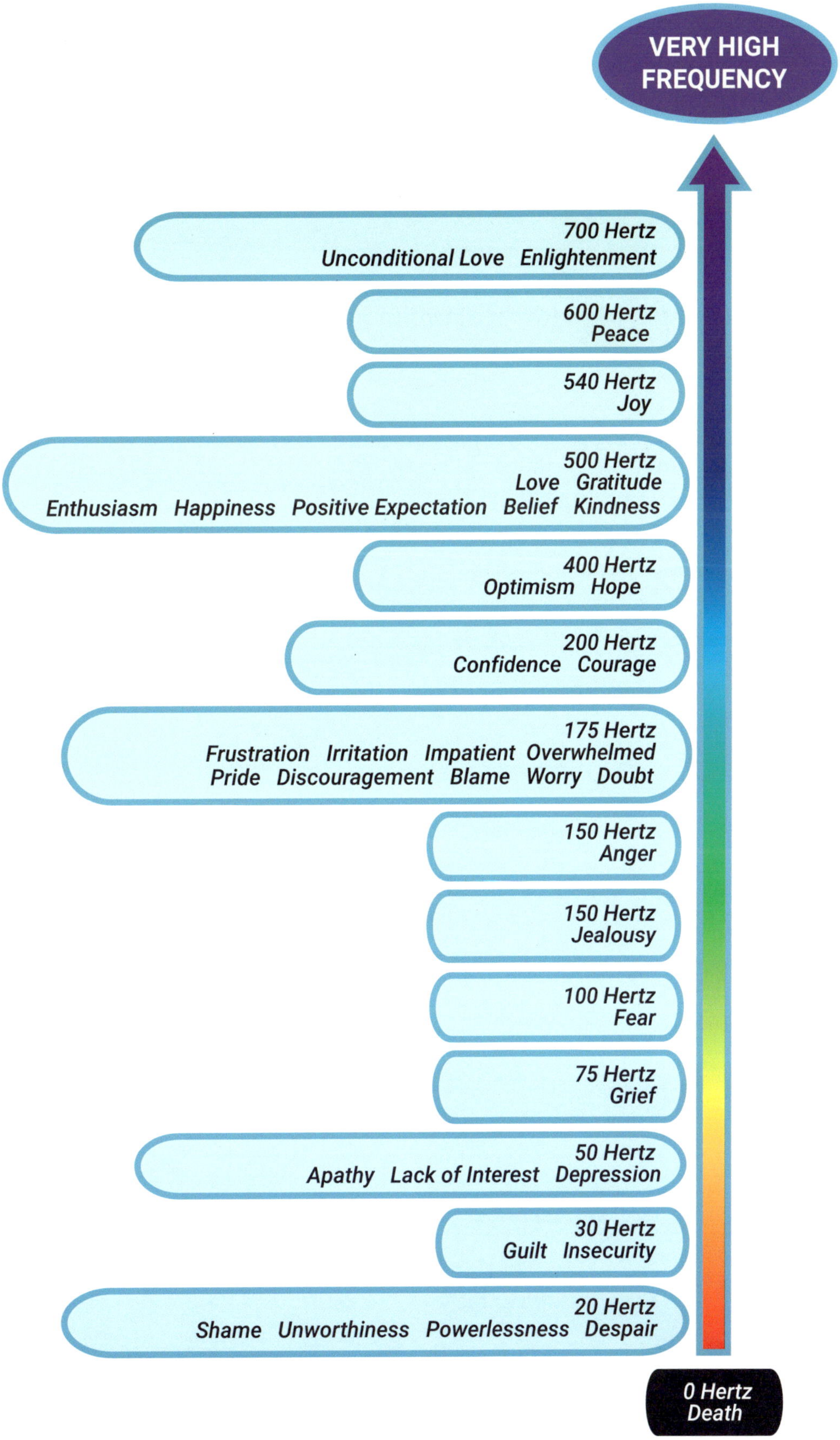
VERY HIGH FREQUENCY
700 Hertz
Unconditional Love Enlightenment
600 Hertz
Peace
540 Hertz
Joy
500 Hertz
Love Gratitude
Enthusiasm Happiness Positive Expectation Belief Kindness
400 Hertz
Optimism Hope
200 Hertz
Confidence Courage
175 Hertz
Frustration Irritation Impatient Overwhelmed
Pride Discouragement Blame Worry Doubt
150 Hertz
Anger
150 Hertz
Jealousy
100 Hertz
Fear
75 Hertz
Grief
50 Hertz
Apathy Lack of Interest Depression
30 Hertz
Guilt Insecurity
20 Hertz
Shame Unworthiness Powerlessness Despair
0 Hertz
Death

What are the emotions that you feel most often? What triggers them? What do you normally do when you have negative feelings which cause lower frequency?

> "Remember that we cannot allow our negative feelings to overcome our effort, progress, and commitment. Negative feelings are acid and positive feelings are alkaline. Cancer does not grow in an alkaline body."

Now that you know how your emotions can affect your body's energy frequency,
What are some things that you can do to help your body's energy frequency to increase?

BALANCE EVERYTHING IN YOUR LIFE

"He gives strength to the weary and increases the power of the weak." - Isaiah 40:29

CANCER BEGINS

Severe Trauma Shock often occurs 1½ to two years before cancer becomes detectable.[3]

See a partial list of some Shock Traumas below. This could be a divorce, death of a loved one, surgery, or other trauma that affects the immune system, shutting down melatonin production, affecting sleep and the regulation of hormones.

EXAMPLE OF SEVERE SHOCK TRAUMA

PSYCHOLOGICAL

- Loss of Home
- Prolonged Anxiety
- Stress
- Dental Visit
- Scary Movies
- Near Drowning
- Nightmares
- Phobias
- Rape or Sexual Assault
- Vaccination
- War Trauma (PTSD)
- Abuse: Domestic, Spousal, Satanic Ritual or any other abuse
- Witness/Participant:
  Death
  Horrific Accident
  Murder
  Violence

EMOTIONAL/MENTAL

- Financial Hardship or Job Loss
- Pregnancy and Birth
- Birth of a sibling
- False Accusation
- Public Speaking
- Suicidal Thoughts
- Potential Loss, Death, or Life-Threatening Illness of close relative or friend
- School Stress
- Being made to write with less dominant hand
- Starting School
- Changing Schools
- Loneliness
- Ostracization
- Divorce

NUTRITIONAL ***(DEFICIENCY OR EXCESS)***

- Minerals
- Vitamins
- Protein
- Fat
- Junk Food Diet
- MTHFR gene
- Hypoglycemia
- Hyperglycemia
- Obesity

Hydration
- Dehydration
- Edema

BIOCHEMICAL

- Infection:
  - Bacterial
  - Virus
  - Fungus
  - Parasite
- Chemical Poisoning:
  - Dioxins
  - PCB's
  - Pesticides
  - Volatile Organic Compounds
  - Fungicides
  - Fertilizer
  - Phthalates
- Toxic Metals:
  - Mercury (teeth anagrams)
  - Lead
  - Copper
  - Fluoride
  - Chemotherapy
  - Nickel
  - Tin
  - Bromine
  - Arsenic
  - Vanadium
  - Strontium
  - Aluminum
  - Gold
  - Silver
  - Iodine

ENVIRONMENTAL

- Weather Related:
  - Cyclone
  - Earthquake
  - House/forest fire
  - Hurricane
  - Flooding
  - Tornado
  - Global Warming
- Electromagnetic Fields
- Radiation
- Pollution
- Plastic Food Storage Bags
- Carbon Monoxide Poisoning
- Home Toxins:
  - Cell Phone
  - Cell Phone Towers
  - Noise (traffic, electric hum, sirens)
  - Wi-Fi (5G will be toxic to us all)

PHYSICAL/STRUCTURAL *(INCLUDING ANYTHING INVASIVE)*

- Bariatric Surgery Procedures including:
  - Gastric Bypass
  - Sleeve gastrectomy
  - Adjustable gastric band
  - Biliopancreatic diversion w/ duodenal switch
  - Roux-en-Y gastric bypass
  - Laparoscopic adjustable gastric banding
- Falls
- Sprains
- Severe or Chronic Disease
- Operations
- Accidents such as ankle sprains, sports injuries, car, bike, motorcycles, etc
- Burns (i.e. Sunburn)
- Concussion
- Dental work
- Scar
- Tattoo
- Genes
- Epigenetic Causes of Illness
- Inflammation
- Mammogram; Breast Ultrasound; Augmentation

*This is only a partial list.

> "The Immune System must be protected above anything else, as it is the only system that heals the body.

Remember: If you are not doing anything to stop the cancer, you are doing something to help it grow.
Do not feed the Beast. Do not eat sugar.

Have you experienced any severe shock or traumas?

Use the last two pages to identify what type of shock or traumas you may have experienced. Feel free to journal your experience and reflect how that shock or trauma has affected you.

What steps have you taken to overcome and heal from those experiences?

> Cancer treatment is like an onion. We must peel off each layer, correct them, and then move down to the next layer to correct these; and, by doing so, we have a chance to heal.

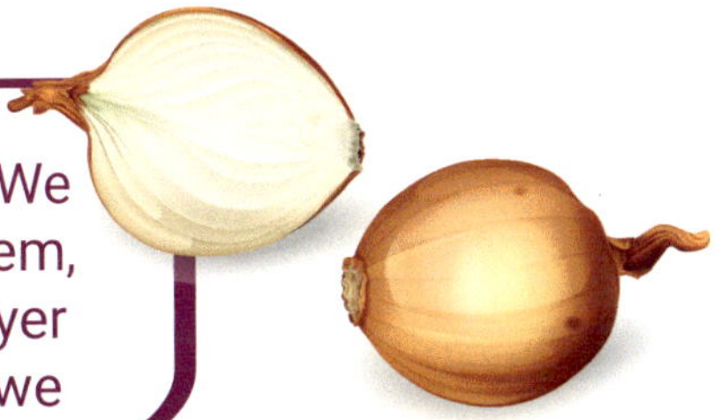

Remember: If you are not doing anything to stop the cancer, you are doing something to help it grow.
Do not feed the Beast. Do not eat sugar.

REPLACE EVERYTHING THAT IS MISSING

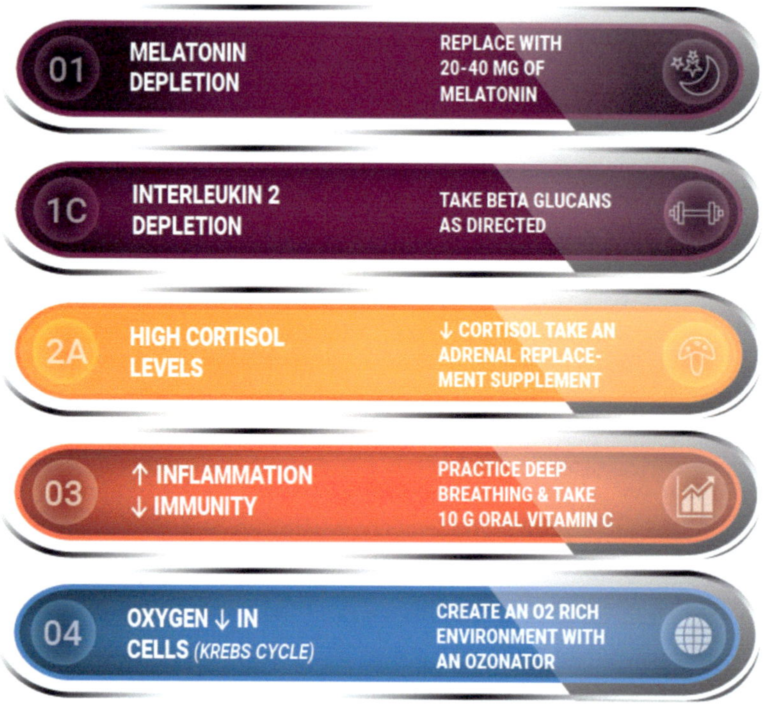

Step 1: Replace melatonin – take 10-40 mg at bedtime to replace missing melatonin.

Step 1C: Take Beta glucans (mushrooms) as directed.

Step 2: Adrenal gland suppression increases cortisol (high stress hormone). Decrease cortisol with the following:

1. Sleep
2. Exercise
3. Decrease stressful thinking
4. Relax
5. Have fun
6. Develop and maintain healthy relationships
7. Spending time with pets
8. Spirituality
9. Eat a healthy diet
10. Supplements
    - Omega-3 fatty acids
    - Ashwagandha
    - Phosphatidylserine
    - Gingko biloba leaf extract, 500mg
    - Choline bitartrate
    - L-Theanine

Step 2B: Adrenaline levels increased:

1. Diet – follow:
    - Brightly colored vegetables
    - Lean white protein such as fish and chicken
    - Whole grain, gluten-free carbohydrates
2. Sleep
3. Methylated B vitamins
4. Decrease inflammation
5. Supplements as directed:
    - Vitamin D
    - Vitamin C
    - Selenium
    - Magnesium
    - Zinc
6. Hydration - 1/2 body weight in ounces of water plus add ounces of water for anything else you drank.
7. Adaptogenic herbs
    - Licorice root
    - Rehmannia

Step 3: Increased inflammation and decreased immunity causes Interleukin-1 production. Interleukin-1 is a performance-killing cytokine that can cause ill health and inflammation [6]. Beta glucans increase immunity.

Step 4: Cancer cannot grow in an O2-rich environment. Buy an oxygenator for water and drink oxygen rich water. Eat the Budwig breakfast to restore oxygenation to cells.

Journal

Remember: If you are not doing anything to stop the cancer, you are doing something to help it grow.
Do not feed the Beast. Do not eat sugar.

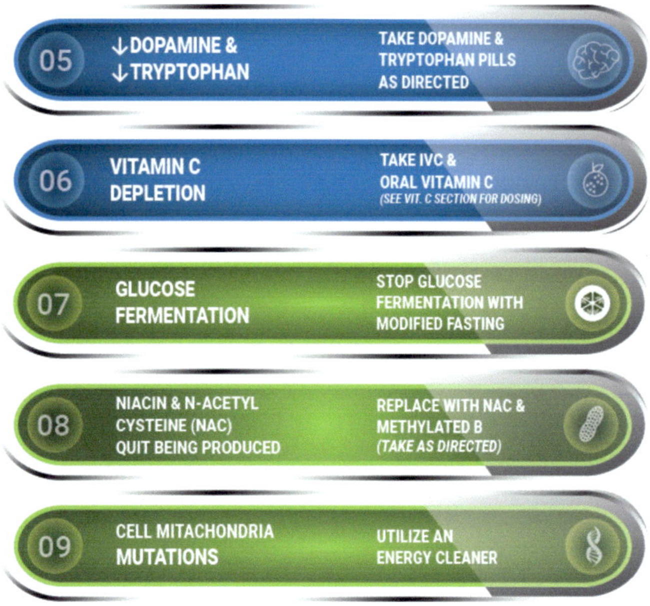

Step 5: Replace dopamine and tryptophan: wear information chips several hours a day to replace levels. Order chips at www.akuRYprodukte.de/en or supplement orally.

Step 6: Vitamin C – both IV and oral. Use caution. Do not use with liver cancer.

Talk to your Oncologist about IV vitamin C. Take oral vitamin C, 12 grams (try crystalline vitamin C to avoid taking 24 500mg pills) in 3 divided doses.[4]

Step 7: Glucose fermentation must be stopped:

Eat cultured foods like yogurt, kefir, kombucha, sauerkraut, kimchi, pickles, sourdough bread, all without sugar. Take Probiotics.

Step 8: Niacin (one of the B vitamins)

Correct this with methylated B vitamins, and N-Acetyl Cysteine (NAC).

Step 9: Cell mitochondrial mutations are decreased as Energy Cleaners decrease deoxyribonucleic acid (DNA) mutations.

Journal

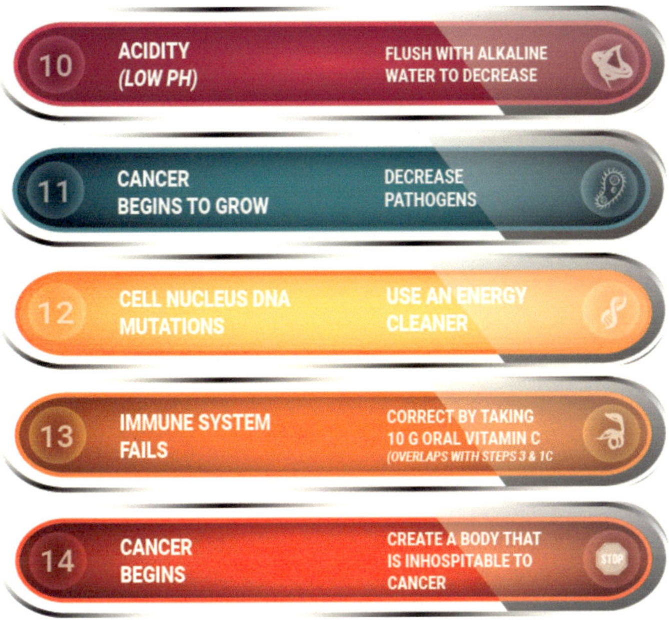

Step 10: Cancer produces lactic acid. Lactic acid causes blood acidity = Decrease Lactic Acid (Acidity) with Alkaline water. Test this with pH strips on both saliva and urine. The goal is to have a reading of each above 7.0. Use baking soda to increase pH. Take 1 teaspoon and stir in 2 ounces of water and drink every two hours until pH tests in the right range. Take calcium lactate or calcium gluconate to decrease the pH and calcium hydroxide or calcium citrate to increase pH. Calcium gluconate to keep it the same.

Step 11: Cancer begins to grow – our bodies harbor vectors and come in contact with them every day on surfaces, in the food we eat, and in the vaccines, and medications we take. Decrease vectors by following a low sugar diet and utilizing the Bob Beck Protocol.

Step 12: Cell nucleus DNA mutations are decreased as Energy Cleaners stop DNA mutations.

Step 13: Immune system starts to fail = Correct Immune system deficiencies with B6, Elderberry, Pelargonium, Olive Leaf Extract, N-Acetyl Cysteine, Astragalus, Larch

Step 14: Cancer cannot grow in a body inhospitable to cancer. In the book you learned how cancer begins and different things that you can do along the way to get rid of it. Let's look at each step and create an implementation plan.

Journal

Remember: If you are not doing anything to stop the cancer, you are doing something to help it grow.
Do not feed the Beast. Do not eat sugar.

ELEVEN NATURAL RECIPES TO ADDRESS CANCER

"Heal me, O Lord, and I will be healed; save me and I will be saved, for you are the one I praise."
- Jeremiah 17:14

01 IV VITAMIN C
Vitamin C is an essential nutrient critical to the healing process.

02 WATER FASTING
If All Else Fails – QUIT EATING!

03 MODIFIED FASTING DIETS (MFDS)
Including Breuss Cancer Cure Diet, Budwig Diet, Ketogenic Diet, Intermittent Fasting, Raw Vegan Diet, Green Drink Fast, and the Epigenetic Diet.

04 HYPERTHERMIA & COLEY'S TOXINS
How immunotherapy heals the body.

05 ELECTRICITY & FREQUENCIES
Sound, light, and electrical energy fields heal the body.

06 BLACK SEED OIL FROM TURMERIC
Antioxidant and anti-inflammatory properties.

07 ALKALINE WATER & BAKING SODA
Cancer cannot grow in an Alkaline environment.

08 PAO PEREIRA & RAUWOLFIA VOMITORIA[7]
Both efficient and non-toxic.

09 FENBENDAZOLE, TURMERIC AND CBD OIL
Fenbendazole is a broad spectrum benzimidazole anthelmintic used against gastrointestinal parasites.

10 OXALIC ACID
Cleanses the blood.

11 BEE VENOM
The anti-cancer agents are melittin and phospholipase.

Did you know that there were so many options available to help you on your journey? Journal what and how you decide to implement them into your program.

> “Time management is critical in any cancer-fighting plan, as there will be multiple steps that must be combined to create the synergy needed to stop the cancer from growing. Doctors’ appointments must be scheduled, meals cooked (these need to be as organic as possible) supplements and nutraceuticals must be taken on schedule, medicines taken as needed, exercise scheduled, and IVs managed. This is in addition to work, home duties, children, and relatives.”

01 IV VITAMIN C

How did you feel after the IV vitamin C administration?

Treatment Volume of Ascorbic Acid	Solution Volume		Withdraw from Solution and Discard	Remaining Solution	Inject Volume of AA into Solution	Inject Volume of $MgCl_2$ into Solution	Final Volume	Infusion Rate	Total Infusion Time
	Ringer Lactate	Sterile Water							
15 grams (30cc)	250cc		31cc	219cc	30cc	1cc	250cc	0.5 - 1.0 g/min	~0.5 h
25 grams (50cc)	500cc		51cc	449cc	50cc	1cc	500cc	0.5 - 1.0 g/min	~1 h
50 grams (100cc)		500cc	102cc	398cc	100cc	2cc	500cc	0.5 - 1.0 g/min	~1.5 h
75 grams (150cc)		750cc	152cc	598cc	150cc	2cc	750cc	0.5 - 1.0 g/min	~2.5 h
100 grams (200cc)		1000cc	202cc	798cc	200cc	2cc	1000cc	0.5 - 1.0 g/min	~3.5 h

“This diet is not applicable for people with low weight or a BMI less than 21. Metformin decreases blood sugar.

Day 1

Day 2

Day 3

Day 4

Day 5

Day 6

Day 7

Remember: If you are not doing anything to stop the cancer, you are doing something to help it grow.
Do not feed the Beast. Do not eat sugar.

02 WATER FASTING

When you are ready to do your water fast, please follow the tips bellow. Write here your plan of action. Please journal your experience. How did you feel?

Remember this is the cheapest diet because all you do is drink water and no food.

WATER FASTING TIPS

① PLANNING

Arrange your schedule. If possible, take time off work. Decide on a length of time for your water fasting cancer cleanse. Fasts can be done for any length of time up to about a month.

You may consider a supervised water fast at a fasting clinic. They can do tests to monitor your health and help ease you back to solid foods.

② REST FREQUENTLY

Fasting is a time for rest. The body will want to sleep more than usual. Listen to your body; you may need 12 hours or more of sleep each night, and naps during the day. Dr. JoAnna Budwig of the Budwig Diet believed rest was imperative to regaining health.

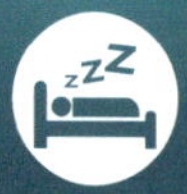

③ DIFFICULTY

The first 3 days are going to be the worst as the cells open up and dispel all the toxins they have stored over the years. Symptoms you may experience could be hunger, irritability, headache, or disorientation. Fortunately, your body is resilient and should quickly adapt. You should start feeling better around the third or fourth day. Many people even report a feeling of euphoria at this point.

④ BREAKING THE FAST

Break your fast slowly. Start by drinking only juices and detox waters, then broths, and gradually add in solid foods. Breaking the fast can be a multi-day process.

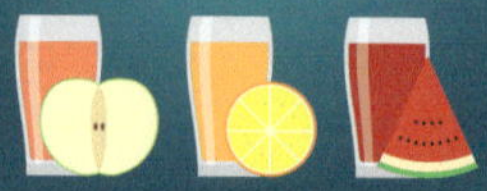

MONDAY

TUESDAY

WEDNESDAY

THURSDAY

FRIDAY

SATURDAY

SUNDAY

Remember: If you are not doing anything to stop the cancer, you are doing something to help it grow.
Do not feed the Beast. Do not eat sugar.

03 MODIFIED FASTING DIETS (MFD)

This section we will be focusing on different types of diets, how they make you feel and meal planning. Use this page to take notes on things you've learned and want to implement.

What do you normally eat? Journal a few days of regular eating, write down what you ate and how you felt throughout the day, moods, physical reactions, etc.

Today's Date:

Breakfast

Drinks & Snacks

☐ ____________________

☐ ____________________

☐ ____________________

☐ ____________________

☐ ____________________

☐ ____________________

Lunch

Dinner

Today I Am Feeling...

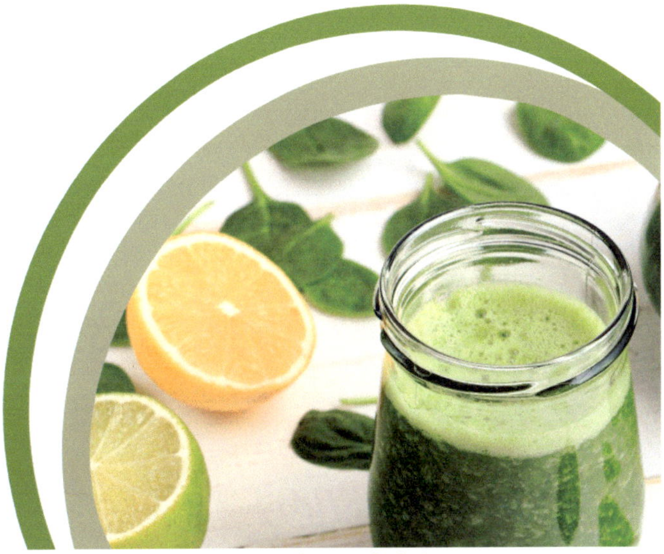

Remember: If you are not doing anything to stop the cancer, you are doing something to help it grow.
Do not feed the Beast. Do not eat sugar.

Today's Date:

Breakfast

Lunch

Dinner

Today I Am Feeling...

Drinks & Snacks

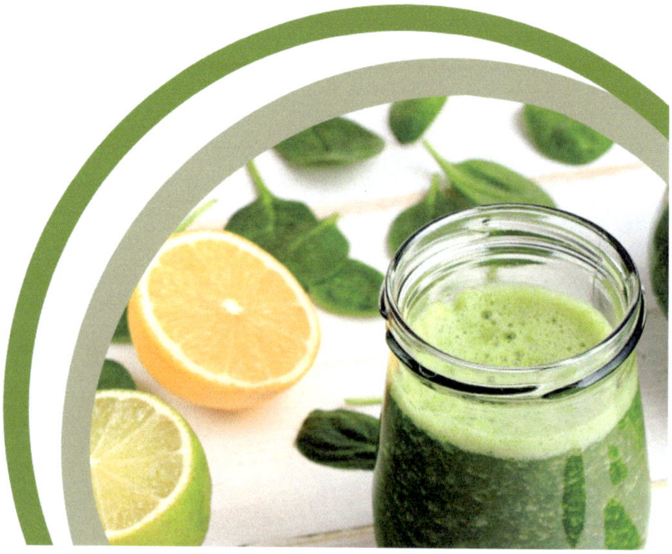

Today's Date:

Breakfast

Lunch

Dinner

Today I Am Feeling...

Drinks & Snacks

- ☐ ______
- ☐ ______
- ☐ ______
- ☐ ______
- ☐ ______
- ☐ ______

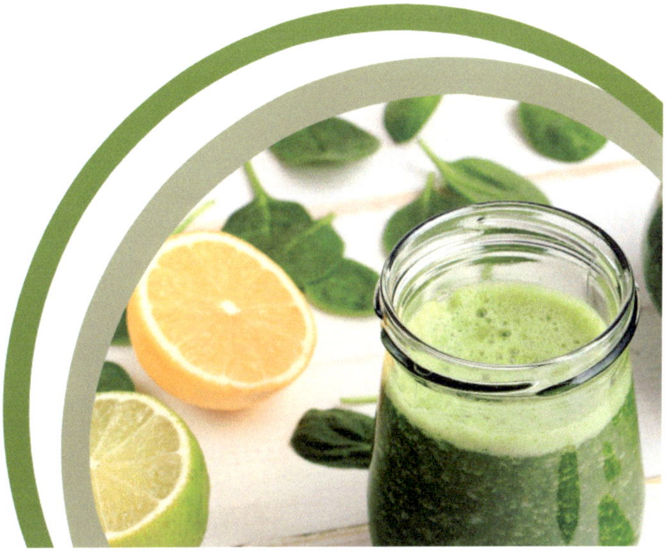

Remember: If you are not doing anything to stop the cancer, you are doing something to help it grow.
Do not feed the Beast. Do not eat sugar.

Today's Date:

Breakfast

Drinks & Snacks

Lunch

Dinner

Today I Am Feeling...

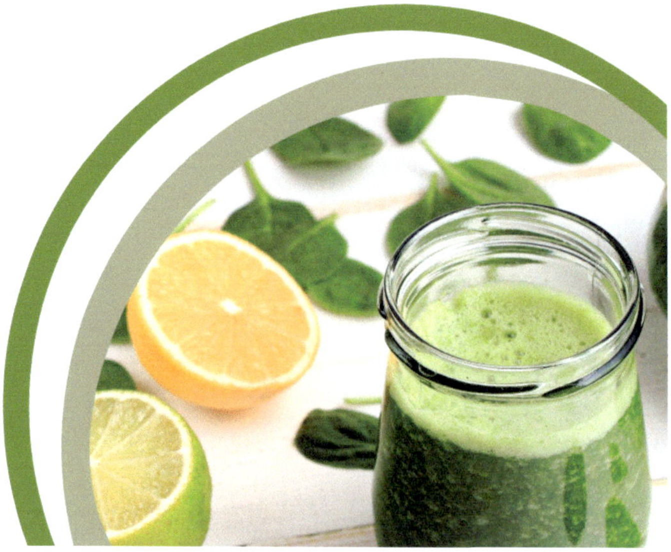

Today's Date:

Breakfast

Lunch

Dinner

Today I Am Feeling...

Drinks & Snacks

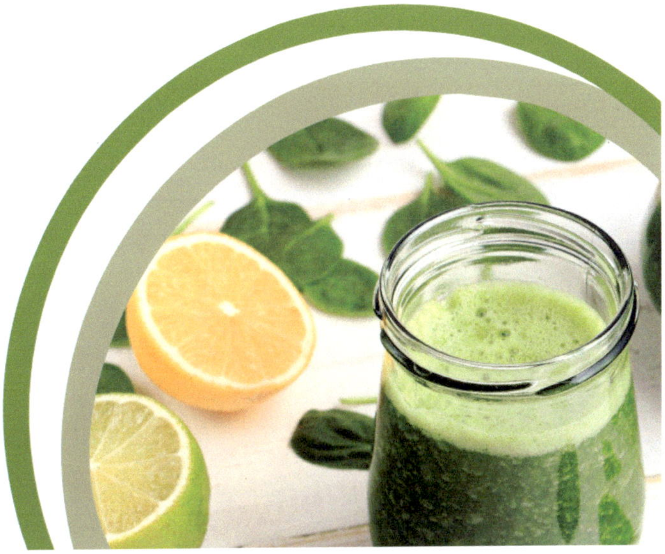

Remember: If you are not doing anything to stop the cancer, you are doing something to help it grow.
Do not feed the Beast. Do not eat sugar.

Today's Date:

Breakfast

Lunch

Dinner

Today I Am Feeling...

Drinks & Snacks

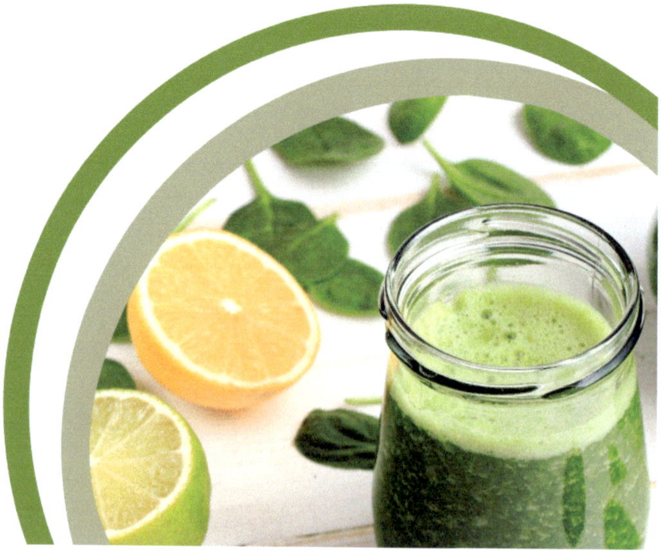

Today's Date:

Breakfast

Lunch

Dinner

Today I Am Feeling...

Drinks & Snacks

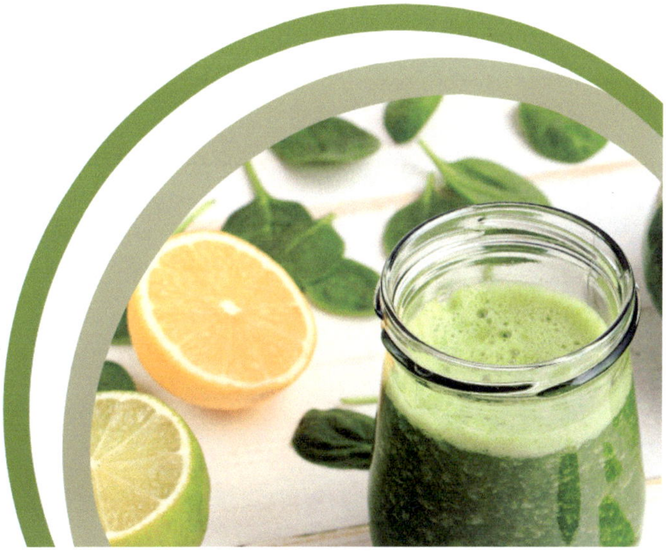

Remember: If you are not doing anything to stop the cancer, you are doing something to help it grow.
Do not feed the Beast. Do not eat sugar.

What did you notice? What are the foods that you felt good afterwards and the ones that did not make you feel good? What foods satisfied you best?

The Budwig Diet

1. Grind 1Tbsp flaxseed. Pour in a bowl.
2. Mix 4 Tbsp of organic ***cottage cheese*** and 2 Tbsp of ***flaxseed oil*** with a wood or plastic spoon in a blender, you can thin it down with a little flax milk, coconut milk, or almond milk (but no other milk).

2. Turn the blender on and blend until the flaxseed oil and cottage cheese are completely blended together. The consistency will be like yogurt and make sure no flaxseed oil is floating on the sides of the blender.

3. Pour over ***ground flaxseeds*** in the bowl. You can add **cinnamon, Stevia, berries, walnuts, almonds, or macadamia nuts, garlic, cayenne, red pepper, or champagne.**

4. Wait 5 minutes for the chemical reaction to complete, then eat within 15 minutes.

The Budwig Diet + Cellect or Trican Powder = BALANCE FATS

Ingredients:

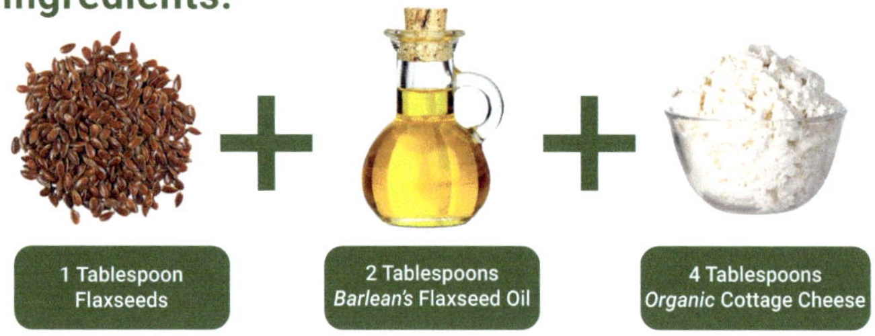

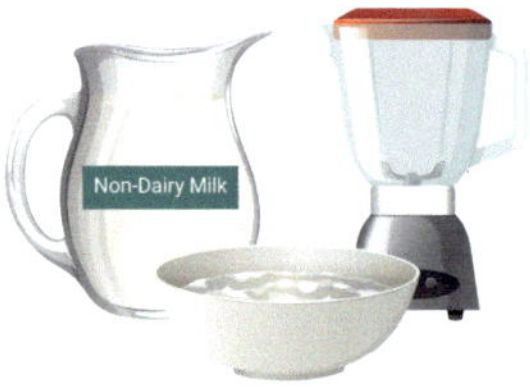

The Budwig mixture should be taken once or twice a day. It should be stirred with a *wooden or plastic spoon*. Wood is ideal and metal should never be used.

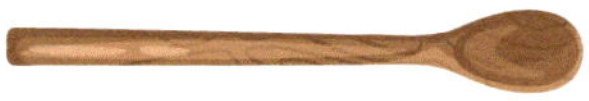

Note #1: Do not take the product Cellect or Trican and the Budwig Diet products within one and a half hours of each other!!

Note #2: Cellect or Trican should be taken immediately before a meal (to prevent stomach upset) and the cod liver oil should be taken during the meal.
This ensures the cod liver is not taken within an hour and a half of the Budwig portion!!

http://cellect.org/order.php
https://www.lifeintegrativemed.com/trican-plain

After reading about different types of diets and fasting, which one do you think works for you? Why?

How are you going to implement it today?

Remember: If you are not doing anything to stop the cancer, you are doing something to help it grow.
Do not feed the Beast. Do not eat sugar.

THE KETO FLU

The keto flu occurs when individuals have not properly detoxed or have been receiving chemotherapy or radiation and have a buildup of heavy metal poisoning or toxins.

BLUNTING HUNGER ON THE KETO DIET

Bringing your body into ketosis virtually eliminates hunger. Once the ketone levels start to rise, the appetite begins to decrease.[19] As long as the body is burning ketones there is no significant energy decrease nor decrease in overall wellbeing. Some people may complain of being tired initially, but this dissipates over time. The brain burns ketones as efficiently as it does carbohydrates. The entire body can run quite effectively on ketones.

SIGNS & SYMPTOMS

Dehydration, headaches, constipation, diarrhea, brain fog, light headedness, electrolyte imbalance, palpitations, muscle cramps, fatigue, metabolic acidosis, and keto rash.

CALORIE RESTRICTION & DIETARY LIMITS

Overall calorie restriction is eating less of everything which is critical for cancer prevention.

1. **Set** carbohydrate **limit at 12-25 carbs daily**
2. **Set** protein **limit at 1.0 protein/kg of lean body mass daily (3 servings a week of red meat)**
3. No alcohol **for three weeks then one glass of red wine. (White wine has NO therapeutic effect or health benefit, as is the same as drinking vodka and kool-aid.)**

> The Keto diet is not applicable for people with low weight or a BMI less than 21%.

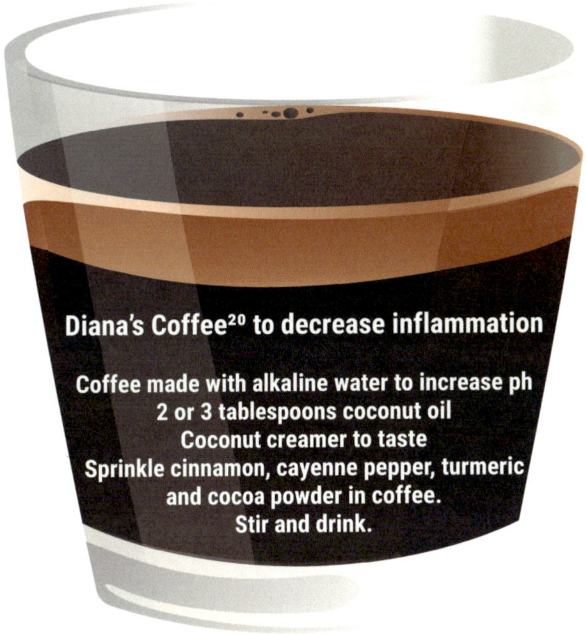

SNACK IDEAS

Try to combine fiber and protein to satisfy your hunger.

1. Celery with almond or walnut butter, or cheese cubes.
2. Cherry tomatoes stuffed with mozzarella cheese.
3. Veggies with hummus.
4. Deviled eggs made with veganaise instead of mayonnaise.
5. Guacamole- stuffed cherry tomatoes.

APPLE CIDER VINEGAR

You must consume 2 tablespoons Apple Cider Vinegar every day as ACV Tea:

1 cup of water with 2 tablespoons Apple Cider Vinegar, 4 drops of lemon essential oil or 1/2 of lemon (juiced), dash of cayenne pepper and maple syrup only to sweeten as a kidney cleanse.

Or use Apple Cider Vinegar as a salad dressing or on vegetables.

INTERMITTENT FASTING

Intermittent fasting is going from 12 to 36 hours without food. Intermittent fasting is not eating breakfast or eating until lunch then eating supper within 6-8 hours while avoiding eating anything 3 hours before bed and not eating sugar until lunch.

Raw Vegan Diet

1. No meat, dairy, wheat, eggs, processed sugar, or alcohol.
2. Eat plenty of fresh fruit, raw vegetables, and drink fresh juice & green smoothies.
3. Drink at least half your weight in ounces of water, plus water for any other drink that is consumed. Example: For a 100 pound person they would drink 50 ounces plus add any additional ounces for anything else they drink.
4. You can drink warm tea and warm water with lemon.

RAW VEGAN DIET

According to Chris Wark, author of *Chris Beat Cancer*, the nutritional value in the food industry is decimated or destroyed.

GREEN JUICE FAST

Start with 3 cups alkaline water and add 3 cups greens, blend until liquified. Then add all other vegetables, including an avocado or MCT oil. Open your spice cabinet and add ½ teaspoon cinnamon, ½ teaspoon cayenne, 1 teaspoon turmeric and ½ teaspoon Celtic salt. These spices decrease inflammation.

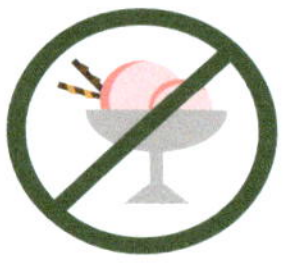

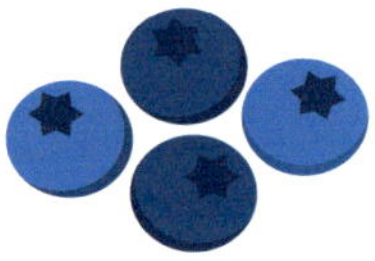

Journal

Remember: If you are not doing anything to stop the cancer, you are doing something to help it grow.
Do not feed the Beast. Do not eat sugar.

Important Note:

Processed food is junk food. Most of us think of junk food as soft drinks, candy, snacks, fast food, and TV dinners. But in reality, junk food is almost any food that has been altered by man and packaged for resale. The best nutrition advice I've ever heard is this:

"If man made it, don't eat it."
– Jack LaLane

Journal

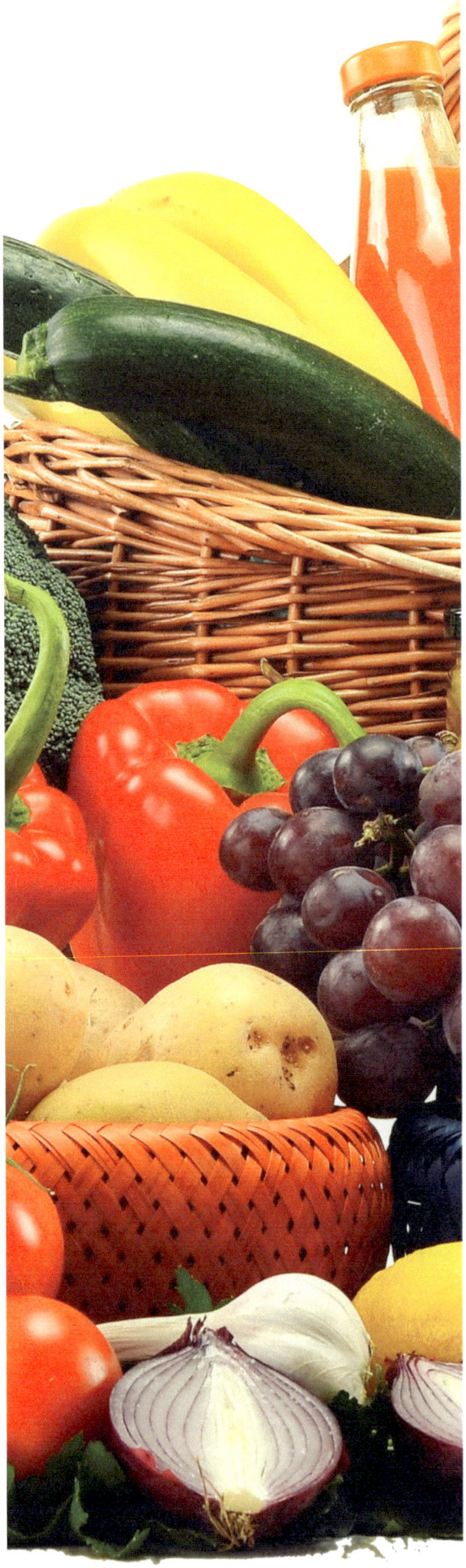

CLEAN EATING

HEALTHY FIVE DAY MEALS

M/W/F

BREAKFAST

Mushroom omelette, fresh strawberries, cottage cheese, freshly squeezed fruit juice

LUNCH

Chef salad, turkey bacon, fruit smoothie

DINNER

Salmon, dill sauce, asparagus, protein powder, snap peas

T/TH

BREAKFAST

Turkey bacon, chicken scramble, freshly squeezed fruit juice

LUNCH

Chicken salad, salad greens, vegetable soup, protein powder

DINNER

Halibut, honey sauce, quinoa, snap peas, zucchini, garlic chicken

WEEKLY MEAL & WATER TRACKER

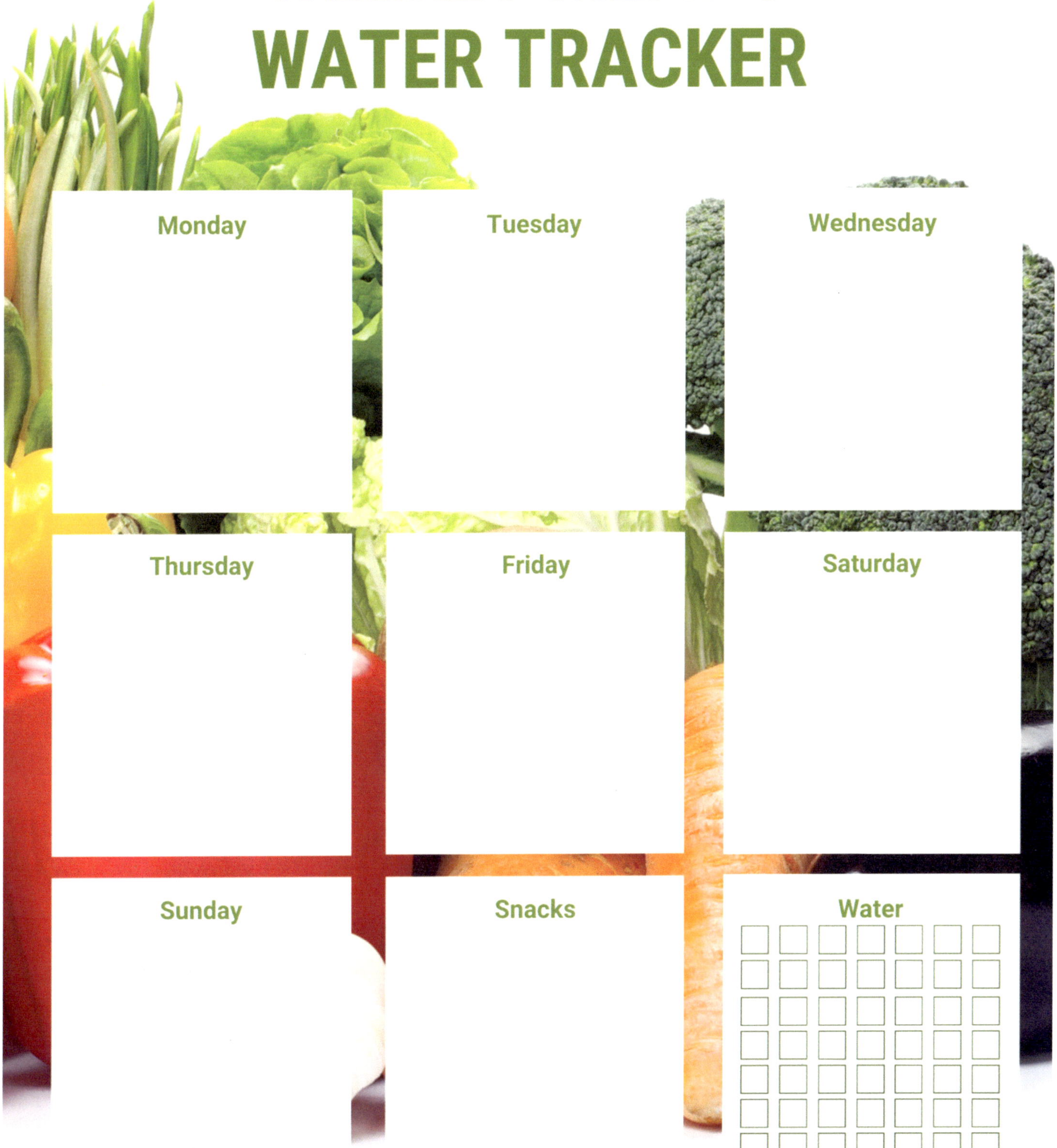

Monday

Tuesday

Wednesday

Thursday

Friday

Saturday

Sunday

Snacks

Water

Remember: If you are not doing anything to stop the cancer, you are doing something to help it grow.
Do not feed the Beast. Do not eat sugar.

WEEKLY MEAL & WATER TRACKER

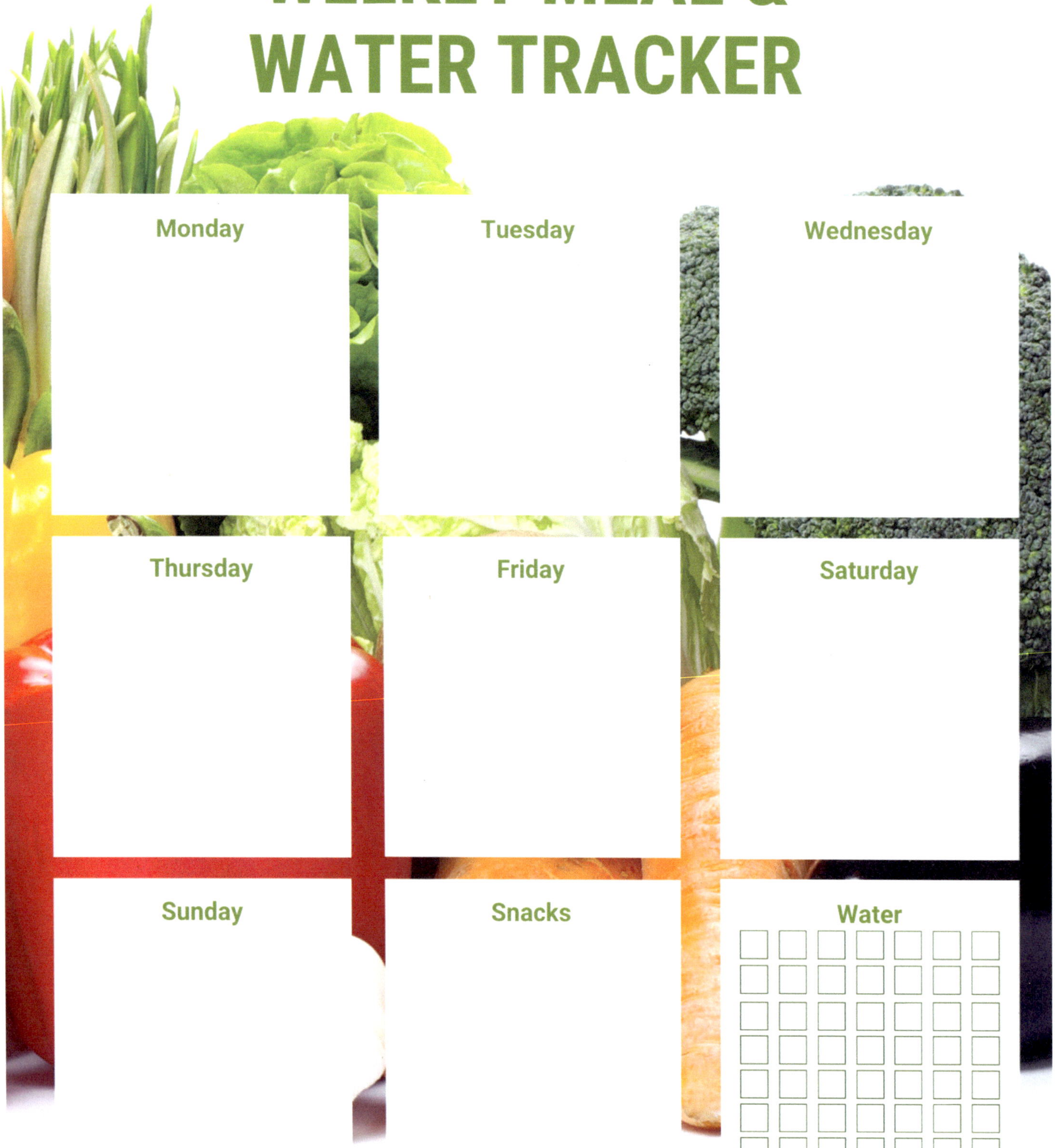

Monday

Tuesday

Wednesday

Thursday

Friday

Saturday

Sunday

Snacks

Water

WEEKLY MEAL & WATER TRACKER

Monday

Tuesday

Wednesday

Thursday

Friday

Saturday

Sunday

Snacks

Water

☐ ☐ ☐ ☐ ☐ ☐ ☐
☐ ☐ ☐ ☐ ☐ ☐ ☐
☐ ☐ ☐ ☐ ☐ ☐ ☐
☐ ☐ ☐ ☐ ☐ ☐ ☐
☐ ☐ ☐ ☐ ☐ ☐ ☐
☐ ☐ ☐ ☐ ☐ ☐ ☐
☐ ☐ ☐ ☐ ☐ ☐ ☐
☐ ☐ ☐ ☐ ☐ ☐ ☐

Remember: If you are not doing anything to stop the cancer, you are doing something to help it grow.
Do not feed the Beast. Do not eat sugar.

Have you used any of the machines mentioned in the book? What was your experience?

Human Body Energy Frequencies

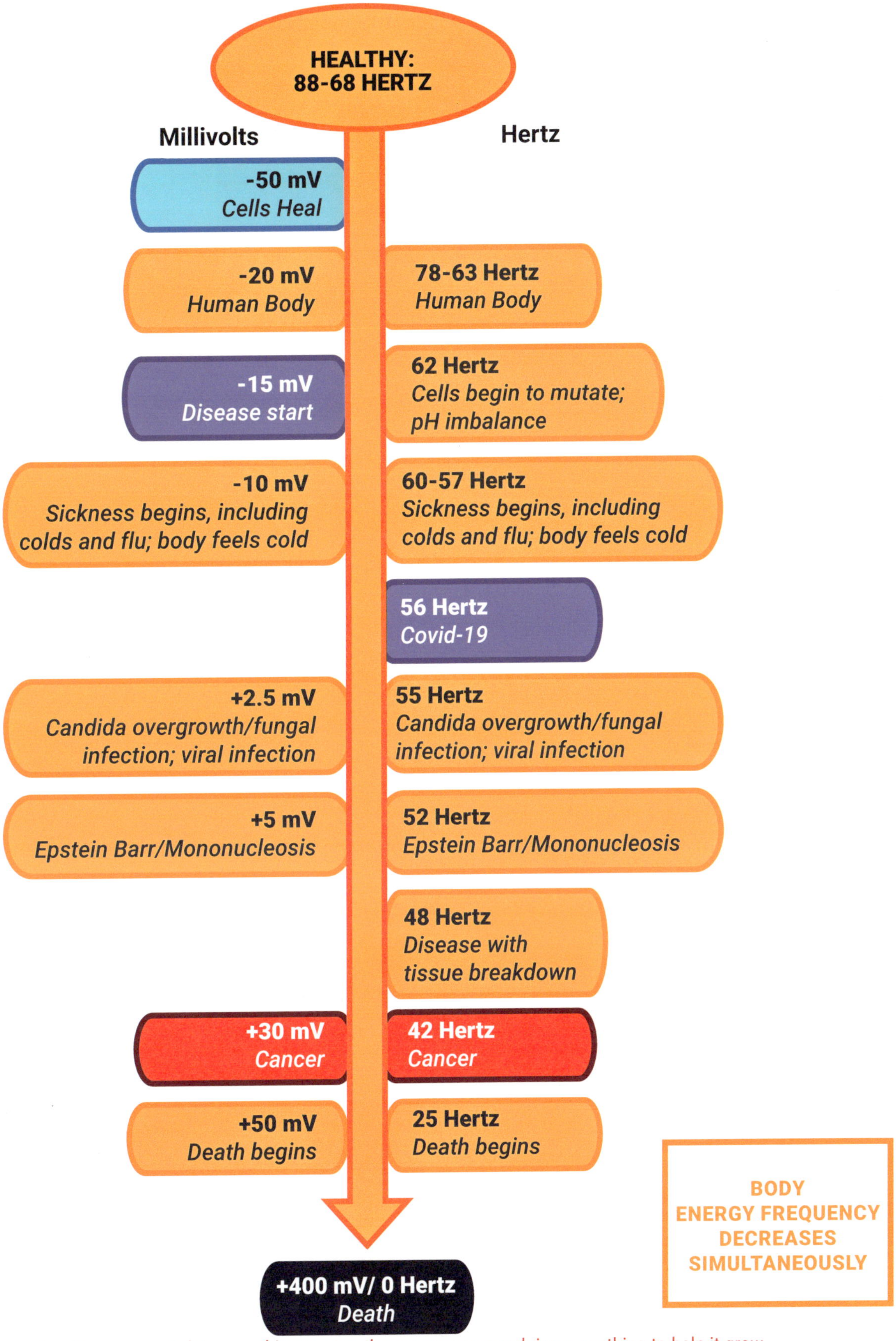

Remember: If you are not doing anything to stop the cancer, you are doing something to help it grow. Do not feed the Beast. Do not eat sugar.

The Baking Soda Recipe to Raise pH

Day 1: Mix 1 teaspoon of baking soda with 1 teaspoon of molasses in a cup of water. Take it once a day for 4 days.

Day 3: Test the saliva with pH strips. The saliva pH should read 7.0 and the urine pH should read higher, at between 7.3 and 7.5.

Day 5: Start taking the solution twice a day.

Days 6 – 10: Take 2 teaspoons each of baking soda and molasses, twice daily. Test the saliva with pH strips on day 10.

> **Stay Alkaline! Cancer cannot grow in an Alkaline environment. For healing the pH has to be 7.88.**

Journal

Journal

To make Baking Soda mixed with Maple Syrup:

Mix 90 teaspoons of maple syrup with 30 teaspoons of baking soda.

The maple syrup must be boiled down to become thicker (the color of caramel). Then the baking soda is added and stirred for 5 minutes until it is fully dissolved.

This preparation should provide about ten days worth of the baking soda remedy. 5 – 7 teaspoons per day is the recommended dose for cancer patients.

Remember: If you are not doing anything to stop the cancer, you are doing something to help it grow.
Do not feed the Beast. Do not eat sugar.

DEEP BREATHING

"Practicing a regular, mindful breathing exercise can be calming and energizing and can even help with stress-related health problems ranging from panic attacks to digestive disorders."
- Andrew Weil, M.D.

Deep Breathing Exercise 4-7-8:[46]

STEP 01
Exhale completely through your mouth, making a whoosh sound.

STEP 02
Close your mouth and inhale quietly through your nose to a mental count of four.

STEP 03
Hold your breath for a count of seven.

STEP 04
Exhale completely through your mouth, making a whoosh sound to a count of eight.

Journal here how you felt after the deep breathing exercise.

09 FENBENDAZOLE, TURMERIC AND CBD OIL

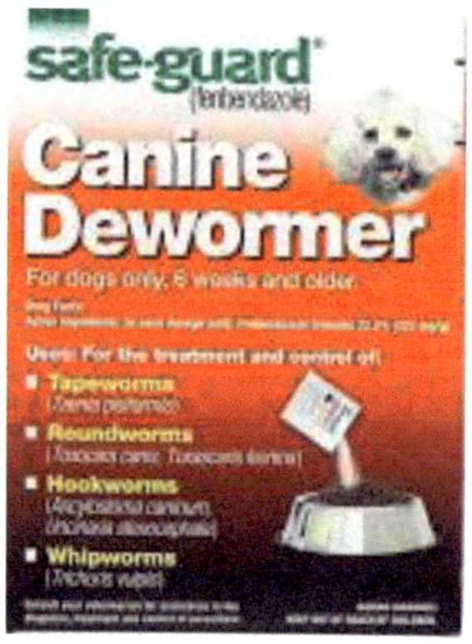

New protocol as of 04/2021:

600mg Fenbedazole twice per day seven days per week plus CBD and Turmeric as directed.

Need to eat a high fat diet or mix dimethyl sulfoxide (DMSO) in it. There are no side effects.

Fenbendazole can be purchased at amazon.com

THE JOE TIPPENS PROTOCOL: FENBENDAZOLE DEWORMER, TURMERIC, AND CBD OIL

MONDAY

TUESDAY

WEDNESDAY

THURSDAY

FRIDAY

SATURDAY

SUNDAY

TRACKER

	M	T	W	T	F	S	S
AM	○	○	○	○	○	○	○
PM	○	○	○	○	○	○	○

Journal daily here how you feel during the Joe Tippens protocol.

> "Parasites survive by consuming the nutrients that you need to thrive."

THERAPEUTIC OXALIC ACID SOLUTION FOR SELF-TREATMENT OF DISEASE

The solution is comprised of 300 milligrams (mg) of oxalic acid dihydrate and 600 milliliters (ml) distilled water. You must use the following instructions carefully in preparing the solution.

Journal here your experience with the oxalic acid diet and the solution.

> All ten of the treatments I have discovered for cancer produce Oxalic Acid.

Remember: If you are not doing anything to stop the cancer, you are doing something to help it grow.
Do not feed the Beast. Do not eat sugar.

BIOCHEMICAL DIET

"Worship the LORD your God, and his blessing will be on your food and water. I will take away sickness from among you..." - Exodus 23:25

"Make your body inhospitable to cancer by including additional vitamins and supplement balancers that are necessary."

Maintain a good balance of vitamin D and have it checked by your medical doctor each time lab work is done. A physician from Germany feels that it is difficult for cancer to grow when vitamin D is at a level of 100.

Take vitamin D3 5000IU every day (get into an anticancer range of 86 or above. My experience is your body will stop supporting cancer at vitamin D 86 IU or higher, so get your lab work checked frequently).

Amino acids must be taken every day as you cannot get the proper amino acids through the meat you eat. Some literature says that meat must be limited to starve out cancer, but to heal and absorb all vitamins and supplements, amino acids must be present with vitamin D.

Weekly Supplement Planner

MONDAY

TUESDAY

WEDNESDAY

THURSDAY

FRIDAY

SATURDAY

SUNDAY

SUPPLEMENT TRACKER

	M	T	W	T	F	S	S
Morning	○	○	○	○	○	○	○
Afternoon	○	○	○	○	○	○	○
Night	○	○	○	○	○	○	○

Remember: If you are not doing anything to stop the cancer, you are doing something to help it grow.
Do not feed the Beast. Do not eat sugar.

PHYSICAL

"Come to me, all who are weary and burdened, and I will give you rest. Take my yoke upon you and learn from me, for I am gentle and humble in heart, and you will find rest for your souls. For my yoke is easy and my burden is light." - Matthew 11:28-3

COFFEE ENEMAS FOR COLON AND LIVER DETOX:

Wait FOUR HOURS between enemas at a minimum to give your body time to recover.

Ingredients:

1) Use organic coffee only
2) A plastic bucket
3) 5' tubing
4) A red rubber catheter or a enema bag

How to Prepare a Coffee Enema

Combine 3 tablespoons of organic coffee with one quart of distilled, filtered or bottled water. Use a saucepan of at least 1 1/2 quarts.

Bring mixture to a boil. Continue boiling for 3-5 minutes or until the froth has mostly boiled off.

Cover and simmer for 20 minutes. Then filter through a drip-style filter system. Let cool to room temperature.

It seems much easier to use an enema bucket than the enema bags. Fill the bucket (first closing clip around the plastic tubing) to 32 ounces. The bucket or bag should end up about 3 1/2-4 feet from the ground.

Have a timer, a book and music available.

Then use some sort of lubricant on the tip of the catheter you will insert (this is a soft tube and should not hurt at all).

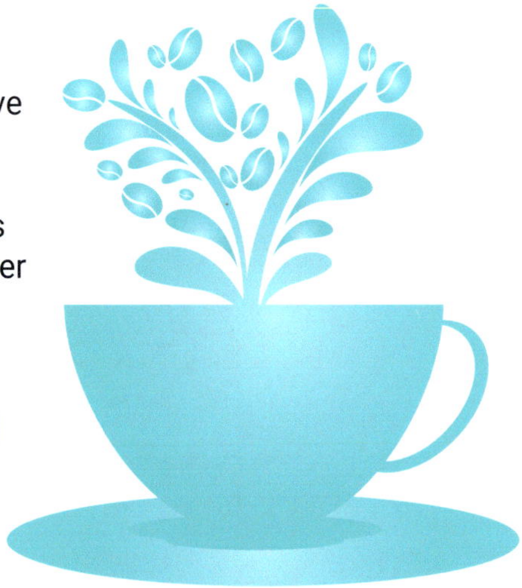

Insert tube and open clip. The coffee will slowly go in as long as you do not have the bucket too high. The higher the bucket, the faster the liquid enters.

Lay on the RIGHT side for this type of enema. Roll onto the knees and forearms to hold it in. Massage the abdomen in a clockwise direction, starting at the lower left and going across and up over the right side, across and then down the left.

Hold it in for 12-15 minutes (that is what the timer is for). Every 3 minutes is a pass thru the liver. It may not be easily done in the beginning, but it is a learned skill. It is usually very relaxing.

Garlic and milk thistle supplements are both good for the colon.
Take as directed.

"RULES FOR DETOXING:

Rule 1: Drink plenty of water.
Rule 2: Detox for 30 days if you have cancer or advanced disease."

Remember: If you are not doing anything to stop the cancer, you are doing something to help it grow.
Do not feed the Beast. Do not eat sugar.

Apple Cider Vinegar Tea

2 tablespoons apple cider vinegar (ACV)

10 drops Lemon essential oil (I use Young Living) or fresh lemon

1 tablespoon maple syrup (no sugar, artificial sweeteners, or honey)

¼ teaspoon cayenne pepper

hot water to fill up the cup

> For those with sensitive stomachs, start slowly with the daily tea and sip small amounts throughout the day. If the stomach is not sensitive, then the tea can be consumed at once. Include the drink in your diet to remove the "sand" in your kidneys so they do not grow larger into stones.

3-Week Protocol

You will need:

- 3 bottles of Citrus Fresh essential oil blend by Young Living
- 1 bottle of Juva Cleanse essential oil blend by Young Living
- 2 bottles of Grapefruit essential oil by Young Living
- 1 bag of empty vegetable capsules

Instructions

- Mix the 3 bottles of Citrus Fresh with the bottle of Juva Cleanse together in a small glass container with a lid.
- Leave overnight
- Pour the contents of the glass container back into the 3 bottles of Citrus Fresh
- You are to use 1 bottle of this mixture every week
- Apply this generously to your target areas. One bottle should be enough for 2 target areas (e.g. stomach and hips) If you have more target areas, you will need more. Do not dilute the oils or it probably won't work.

Take 5-12 drops of Grapefruit, either internally by using a capsule (available at Young Living) or rubbing this on the target areas also.

> Start your day with a cup of hot, clean, apple cider vinegar (ACV) tea before breakfast as this will allow your system to flush away toxins. Wait 2 hours to eat.

EXERCISE – AVOID LACTIC ACID- JUST WALK!
Check daily box bellow and track your exercise.

Monthly Exercise TRACKER

MONTH												TIME	EXERCISE
J	F	M	A	M	J	J	A	S	O	N	D	AM/PM	ACTIVITY

Remember: If you are not doing anything to stop the cancer, you are doing something to help it grow.
Do not feed the Beast. Do not eat sugar.

ESSENTIAL OILS

"Then they cried to the LORD in their trouble, and he saved them from their distress. He sent out his word and healed them: he rescued them from the grave. Let them give thanks to the LORD for his unfailing love and his wonderful deeds for mankind." - Psalms 107:19-21

What essential oils have you use and how? Journal your experience.

"Frankincense and Myrrh are the most used oils for cancer.

> Do not heat oils. Heating these oils destroys their healing properties. It's always best to use a cold diffuser.

Lung Cancer Recipe

Rub on chest wall or in retention enema or use this recipe in a capsule inserted into the rectum:

15 drops Frankincense
5 drops clove
5 drops ravensara
4 drops Myrrh
2 drops sage

EMOTIONS
WHAT YOU BELIEVE CAN KILL YOU

"Surely, he took up our pain and bore our suffering, yet we considered him punished by God, stricken by him, and afflicted. But he was pierced for our transgressions, he was crushed for our iniquities; the punishment that brought us peace was on him, and by his wounds we are healed."
- Isaiah 53:4-5

Today there is a much greater awareness of the relationship between depression and lung cancer, and how both conditions feed into one another on a biochemical level – not just from the trauma associated with a cancer diagnosis and the horrors of conventional treatment. What can you do today to balance your emotional life?

The trick is to restore a healthy methylation cycle and get glutathione back into the cells. What are you doing to start that process?

> Cancer is a disease of the mind, body, and spirit. A proactive and positive spirit is alkalizing and helps the cancer warrior be a survivor. Anger, unforgiveness, and bitterness put the body into a stressful and acidic environment. Learn to have a loving and forgiving spirit. Learn to relax and enjoy life.

Remember: If you are not doing anything to stop the cancer, you are doing something to help it grow.
Do not feed the Beast. Do not eat sugar.

GOOD LUCK!

I'll be in touch via email to see how you're tracking. Please don't hesitate to contact me if you have any questions or need some support along the way.

I'd also love to see photos of your progress! Email me your photos or post your photos or stories on Instagram and tag my profile.

I'm excited to see your results. You got this!

Diana Wright

@DIANAWRIGHT_ND

WWW.DIANAWRIGHTND.COM

INFO@DIANAWRIGHTND.COM

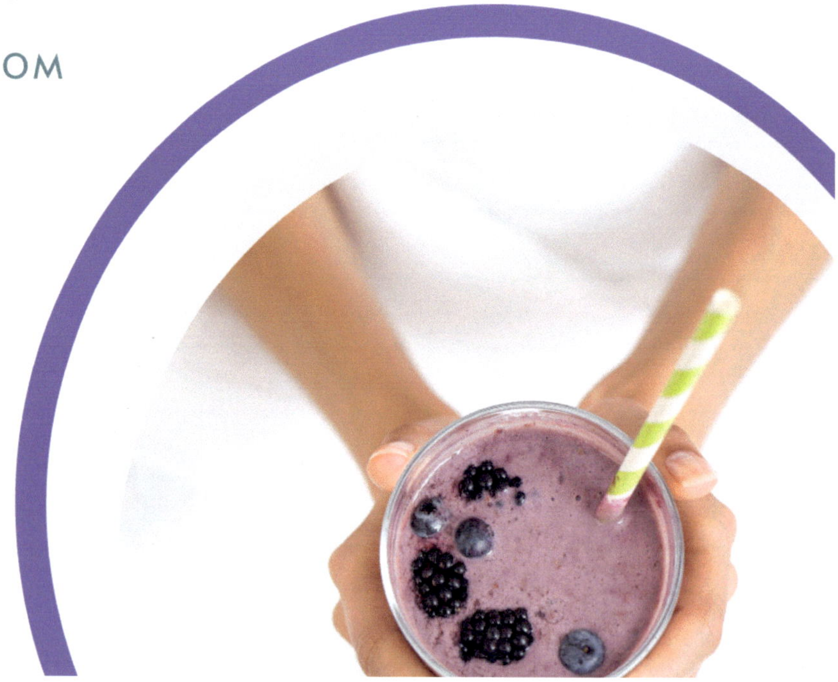

Made in the USA
Las Vegas, NV
09 November 2026

57762019R00045